Eat Well to Live Well

The Essential Guide to Clean Eating and Active Living

DR. NIMI AWORINDE

DEDICATION

To my mum, who nourished me with love. As my first source of nutrition, you are priceless to me.

CONTENTS

INTRODUCTION

In a world full of ever-changing diet trends and conflicting health advice, one thing remains constant: nourishment is key to vitality. Welcome to "Eat Well to Live Well: The Essential Guide to Clean Eating and Active Living," your guide to a life of abundance, energy, and wellness.

This essential book takes you beyond basic sustenance, exploring the power of clean eating and active living. Get ready to discover the secrets to a vibrant life as we delve into nutrition, movement, and holistic well-being.

Eating clean goes beyond a simple diet - it's a lifestyle focused on providing your body with the nutrients it needs to thrive. By choosing whole, healthy foods, you're not only nourishing your body but also your mind. Clean eating is all about making smart food decisions to boost your overall health and wellness.

Active living encourages you to make physical activity a part of your everyday life. You don't need to dedicate hours to the gym; instead, you can discover enjoyable ways to stay active and keep moving all day long.

Living a healthy lifestyle goes beyond simply avoiding sickness; it is about thriving in all aspects of life. When we make our health a priority, we can unleash our true capabilities and enjoy increased energy, improved mental health, and enhanced emotional well-being.

Living healthy helps you live longer, and gives you a sense of fulfillment and happiness. By making conscious choices about what we eat and how we move, we are creating the foundation for a vibrant and rewarding life.

Whether you're a health pro or new to wellness, this book will help you reclaim your health, revitalize your spirit, and embrace a lifestyle where every bite and every step brings you closer to the radiant life you deserve.

Eat Well to Live Well is your essential guide on this life-changing journey. In this book, you'll find practical advice, great meal plans and delicious recipes that are easy to understand, and will help you easily incorporate clean eating and active living in your daily lifestyle.

We'll start by exploring the principles of clean eating, including how to build a healthy and nutritious pantry, plan balanced meals, and make wholesome food choices. Then, we'll dive into active living, giving you tips on how to find the right exercise routines, stay motivated, and include regular physical activity into your daily routine.

This book is more than a guide—it's an empowerment tool. As you embark on this journey, you'll discover how small, consistent changes can cause huge improvements in your health and happiness.

Join me on this journey to unlock the incredible benefits that come from nourishing your body and embracing an active lifestyle.

PART I: UNDERSTANDING CLEAN EATING

1 THE PRINCIPLES OF CLEAN EATING

Clean eating is more than a diet; it's a lifestyle that changes you perception of food, helping you improve your health and overall well-being. It encourages you to eat more whole, natural foods and avoid processed foods, in order to ensure that your diet is as close to natural as possible.

The origin of modern day clean eating can be traced to the early 20th century when food industrialization introduced humans to processed foods.This led to the rise of health-conscious people and groups who began to advocate for the return to natural and unprocessed foods.

The peak of this movement was in the 1960s and 1970s when there was a surge in organic farming and the development of healthy food stores.

However, in recent years the clean eating trend has gained massive popularity. This was driven by increasing awareness of the dangers of processed foods and the merits of natural diets.

Principles of Clean Eating

1. Whole Foods

Whole foods are foods that are unprocessed or minimally processed, which means that they retain their nutrients. Examples of whole foods are fresh fruits and vegetables, grains, nuts and seeds, proteins, and healthy fats.

Whole foods are nutrient-dense, meaning they provide a high amount of vitamins, minerals, compared to their number of calories.

2. Minimal Processing

Minimally processed foods have been altered as little as possible. They contain no or very little refined sugars, artificial ingredients, and preservatives.

The goal of clean eating is to ensure that we eat foods in their most natural and untouched forms. This often means making meals from scratch and avoiding fast food.

3. Nutrient Density

Nutrient density means the amount of nutrients in relation to the number of calories in a particular food. Foods that are nutrient-dense provide a more nutrients with fewer calories.

Examples include leafy green vegetables, berries, nuts, seeds, and lean proteins. Clean eating helps avoid empty calories that contribute to weight gain and harmful diseases.

Advantages of Clean Eating

Adopting clean eating as a lifestyle does not only improve the quality of the food you eat, it enhances your energy levels, helps you manage your weight, improves your gut health, reduce harmful inflammation and improve your mental well-being.

Clean eating also has benefits for the environment. It promotes sustainably sourced, organic foods which ameliorates the harmful environmental impact of food production to individuals and the planet. It benefits individual health, as well as the health of the planet.

———————————

As you continue reading this book, you will learn practical strategies to help you include clean eating into your daily life and create delicious recipes that make healthy eating enjoyable.

2 BUILDING A CLEAN EATING PANTRY

A properly filled pantry is fundamental in the practice of clean eating. One sure way to set yourself up for success is to stock up your pantry shelves with nutritious whole foods and snacks.

In this chapter, you will discover the must-haves in your pantry. You will also learn how to read labels of your foods to avoid hidden additives. We will explore helpful grocery shopping tips and meal planning.

Essential Pantry Staples

For a successful clean eating lifestyle, it is essential to stock your pantry with an array of whole foods. A few examples of staples that must be found in your pantry are:

1. Whole Grains such as brown rice, quinoa, barley, oats, whole grain pasta and flour.

2. Legumes and Beans such as brown beans, black beans, chickpeas, lentils, split peas and other pulses.

3. Nuts and Seeds like almonds, walnuts, chia seeds, and flax seeds, almond butter and peanut butter.

4. Healthy Oils and Fats like extra virgin olive oil, coconut oil, avocado oil, ghee and organic butter.

5. Natural Sweeteners such as raw honey, maple syrup, dates and coconut sugar.

6. Condiments and Sauces, such as mustard, apple cider vinegar, tamari (gluten-free soy sauce), homemade or clean-ingredient sauces and dressings.

7. Herbs and Spices, such as basil, cilantro, and rosemary. Spices like turmeric, cumin, and paprika.

8. Fresh and Dried Fruits, such as apples, bananas, and berries. Unsweetened dried fruits like apricots, raisins, and dates.

By having these staples readily available, not only will you be able to whip up fresh and nutritious meals, but you will also avoid the temptation to snack on unhealthy foods when hungry.

Reading Labels and Avoiding Hidden Additives

It is essential to read and understand food labels in order to make informed choices about the food we eat. A lot of processed foods have additives that may not be so obvious, and can destroy your clean eating lifestyle.

These are the things to look out for on your food labels:

1. Ingredients List

- Shop for products with short and simple ingredient lists with items that can be easily recognized.
- Stay away from items that contain flavors, artificial colors and some preservatives.
- Try to avoid foods containing high-fructose corn syrup, hydrogenated oils, and monosodium glutamate (MSG).

2. Nutrition Facts

- Look out for the serving size and number of servings per container.
- Check the quantity of sodium, sugar, trans and saturated fats

    For reference,
- *Daily sodium intake should be between 1.5-2.3mg.*
- *Daily sugar intake should be less than 30g for adults, 24g for children aged 7-10, and 19g for children 6 and under.*
- *Avoid trans and unsaturated fats as much as possible. They can lead to clogged arteries*

and a myriad of health problems.

3. Hidden Sugars

- There are many synonyms for sugar in ingredient lists, such as sucrose, dextrose, and malt syrup.
- Choose products with few or no added sugars.

4. Additives and Preservatives

- Avoid common additives such as aspartame, sulfites and sodium nitrate.
- Ingredient lists including items such as "natural flavors" should also be avoided, as they are often misleading.

By carefully examining the labels, you can avoid these hidden additives in your food, and choose healthier foods that will aid your clean eating lifestyle.

Tips for Grocery Shopping and Meal Planning

A critical approach to shopping for groceries and planning meals can make your clean eating lifestyle more enjoyable.
These are some tips that can help you:

1.   Plan Your Meals
Set out time to plan your meals weekly. Choose meals that incorporate fresh vegetables and ingredients as

well as your pantry staples.

2.   Create a Shopping List
Before heading to the grocery store, be sure to write out all the ingredients that you need for your recipes. Ensure you follow that list strictly to avoids impulse buying.

3.   Shop the Perimeter
While at the grocery store, shop at the outer aisles of the store where fresh produce and ingredients are usually located. Stay away from the inner aisles which are filled with processed foods.

4.   Buy in Bulk
To save money and avoid wastage, it is better to buy non-perishable staple items such as nuts, beans and grains in bulk. Ensure that the items are stored in airtight containers to preserve their freshness.

5.   Buy Seasonal and Local Produce
Purchase fruits and vegetables while in season. This ensures great tasting and nutritious foods. You can get these at your local store or farmers' market.

6.   Prepare Ahead
As soon as you get home from the store or market, wash and chop the perishable food items to keep them fresh. Cook your proteins and grains in large batches that can be used all week.

These tips will help you reduce your grocery expenditure and food wastage, as well as ensuring you have all you need to eat nutritious meals

3 MEAL PREPARATION AND PLANNING

The importance of planning your meals cannot be overemphasized. By carving out time for meal planning and preparation, you are able to be in control over everything that goes into your body. This is important in ensuring a nutritious, healthy and balanced diet.

Meal planning also helps in the following ways:

1. It Saves Time and Reduces Stress
Having your meals planned out reduces the daily stress of figuring out what to eat for the day, and allows you to focus your energy on other matters.

2. It Ensures Nutritional Balance
Meal planning ensures that you consume a variety of nutrients, which are essential for maintaining your health and energy.

3. It Helps You Avoid Unhealthy Choices

When healthy meals are readily available, it reduces the chances of choosing processed foods.

4. It Aids Portion Control and Reduces Costs
Preparing home made meals enables you to control portion sizes and reduce the cost of eating out frequently.

Weekly Meal Planning Strategies

Regular meal planning requires you to organize your meals and establish a routine. Once you practise this regularly and establish a routine, it will get easier. These strategies can help you begin:

1. Set Aside Time
Allocate a particular time weekly for planning your meals and preparing ingredients. Sundays are a popular choice, however you can select any day that is convenient for you.

2. Create a Meal Time Table
Curate a weekly meal time table that includes three meals and snacks. Take your nutritional needs, medications (if any) and other needs into consideration, and ensure that your meals are balanced.

3. Make a Shopping List
Based on the weekly meal time table you have created, curate your shopping list. Ensure that you stick to the list and avoid impulse purchases.

4. Use Versatile Ingredients
Select ingredients that can be used in various recipes in order to reduce waste and save time.

Sample Meal Plans and Recipes

These are some sample meal plans and recipes that incorporate the principles of clean eating that we previously discussed. They include a wide range of intercontinental ingredients for a diverse and nutritious diet.

Sample Meal Plan

Breakfast
- Monday: Scrambled eggs with sautéed spinach and plantains
- Tuesday: Oatmeal topped with fresh fruits and nuts
- Wednesday: Smoothie with bananas, spinach, and almond milk
- Thursday: Avocado toast on whole-grain bread with a side of yams
- Friday: Greek yogurt with honey, granola, and mixed berries

Lunch
- Monday: Grilled chicken salad with mixed greens,

tomatoes, cucumbers, and a vinaigrette dressing
- Tuesday: Yam and vegetable stir-fry with a side of beans
- Wednesday: Quinoa bowl with roasted sweet potatoes, black beans, and avocado
- Thursday: Mixed vegetable soup with a side of whole-grain bread
- Friday: Grilled fish with steamed broccoli and plantains

Dinner
- Monday: Baked plantains with a side of sautéed greens and grilled shrimp
- Tuesday: Nigerian brown rice jollof with a mixed vegetable salad
- Wednesday: Roasted chicken with sweet potatoes and green beans
- Thursday: Egusi soup with spinach and a side of yams
- Friday: Stir-fried tofu with bell peppers, onions, and a side of brown rice

---

Recipes

Baked Plantains

Ingredients
2 ripe plantains
1 tablespoon olive oil
Salt to taste

Instructions
1. Preheat the oven to 400°F (200°C).
2. Peel and slice the plantains into 1/2-inch thick slices.
3. Massage the plantain slices with olive oil and a pinch of salt.
4. Spread the slices on a baking sheet in a single layer.
5. Bake for 20-25 minutes, turning once, until golden brown.

Nigerian Brown Rice Jollof

Ingredients
3 cups brown rice
1/4 cup vegetable oil
1 large onion (chopped)
2 bell peppers (blended)
2 tomatoes (blended)
3 tablespoons tomato paste
2 cups chicken broth
1 teaspoon thyme
1 teaspoon curry powder
Salt and pepper to taste

Instructions
1. Heat the oil in a large pot over medium heat. Add the onions and cook until translucent.
2. Add the tomato paste and blended bell peppers and tomatoes. Cook for about 5 minutes.
3. Stir in the chicken broth, thyme, curry powder, salt, pepper and then rice.
4. Cover and simmer for 20-25 minutes, or until

the rice is cooked and the liquid is absorbed.
5. Fluff with a fork before serving.

Egusi Soup with Spinach

Ingredients
1 cup ground egusi (melon seeds)
1/2 cup palm oil
1 onion (chopped)
2 tomatoes (blended)
1 pound spinach (washed and chopped)
2 cups chicken broth
1 teaspoon crayfish (optional)
Salt and pepper to taste

Instructions
   1. Heat the palm oil in a large pot over low heat.
Add the onions and cook until soft.
   2. Add the tomatoes and cook for another 5
minutes.
   3. Stir in the ground egusi and cook for 5-7
minutes, stirring constantly.
   4. Add the chicken broth and bring to a boil.
   5. Reduce the heat to low and simmer for 15
minutes.
   6. Add the spinach, crayfish, salt, and pepper.
Cook for another 5-7 minutes until the spinach is
tender.

Baked Lemon Herb Chicken with Roasted Vegetables

Ingredients:
4 boneless, skinless chicken breasts

2 tablespoons olive oil
2 tablespoons fresh lemon juice
2 teaspoons dried oregano
2 teaspoons dried thyme
4 garlic cloves, minced
Salt and pepper to taste

Roasted Vegetables:
2 cups baby carrots
2 cups Brussels sprouts, halved
1 red onion, cut into wedges
2 tablespoons olive oil
Salt and pepper to taste

Instructions:
1. Preheat the oven to 400°F (200°C).
2. In a small bowl, mix together the olive oil, lemon juice, oregano, thyme, minced garlic, salt, and pepper.
3. Place the chicken breasts in a baking dish and pour the mix over them. Let sit for at least 15 minutes.
4. Arrange the baby carrots, Brussels sprouts, and red onion on a baking sheet. Spray with olive oil, and then season with salt and pepper.
5. Place the chicken and vegetables in the oven. Bake for 25-30 minutes, or until the chicken is cooked through and the vegetables are tender and lightly browned.
6. Serve the chicken with the roasted vegetables.

Berry Chia Pudding

Ingredients:
1 cup unsweetened almond milk
1/2 cup mixed berries (blueberries, raspberries, strawberries)
1 tablespoon maple syrup (optional)
1/2 teaspoon vanilla extract

Instructions:
1. In a blender, combine the almond milk and half of the mixed berries. Blend until smooth.
2. Pour the mixture into a bowl and stir in the chia seeds, maple syrup (if using), and vanilla extract.
3. Let the mixture sit for about 10 minutes, then stir again to prevent the chia seeds from clumping.
4. Cover and refrigerate for at least 2 hours or overnight, until thickened.
5. Top with the remaining berries before serving.

4 NUTRITIONAL BALANCE AND PORTION CONTROL

Macronutrients: Proteins, Carbs, and Fats

Proteins

Proteins are important building blocks of the body. They are essential for maintenance, growth and repair of tissues. Good sources of protein are lean meats, poultry, fish, eggs, dairy products, legumes, nuts, and seeds. Each meal should include at least one source of protein.

Carbohydrates

Carbohydrates are the body's main energy source and are important for supporting brain function and physical activity. They come in a number of forms such as sugars, starches, and fiber. Healthy carbohydrate sources are fruits, vegetables, whole grains and dairy products.

Choose complex carbohydrates like whole grains and vegetables, which provide continuous energy and important nutrients. Limit the intake of processed carbohydrates like white bread and sugary snacks.

Fats

Fats are important nutrients required for different functions such as insulation, hormone production and nutrient absorption.

There are two major categories of fats: unsaturated fats (monounsaturated and polyunsaturated) and saturated fats. Unsaturated fats remain the healthiest choice. Some great sources of healthy fats are olive oil, coconut oil, avocados, nuts and seeds.

Micronutrients: Vitamins and Minerals

Vitamins

Vitamins are important micronutrients that have vital functions in metabolism, immunity, and cell function. They are divided into water-soluble (vitamins B and C) and fat-soluble (vitamins A, D, E, and K).

Fill your diet with a range of fruits, vegetables, healthy fats and whole grains to ensure adequate intake and absorption of vitamins. You could also take multivitamin supplements (after consulting your doctor) if you have certain dietary restrictions (e.g vegan) or vitamin deficiencies.

Minerals

Minerals are vital inorganic compounds useful for fluid balance, nerve function and bone health. Examples include iron, calcium, iodine and many others.

Eating a variety of nutrient dense foods such as nuts, seeds, dairy products, leafy greens is a sure way to ensure optimal intake of minerals.

Understanding Portion Sizes and Balanced Meals

Portion Control

It's important to watch your portion sizes in order to keep a healthy weight and get the right nutrients. The specific portion sizes you need may differ based on factors like age, gender, activity level, and metabolism.

As a rule of thumb, try to fill half your plate with fruits and veggies, one-quarter with lean proteins, and one-quarter with whole grains or starchy veggies. Be mindful of portion sizes, especially when eating out or snacking mindlessly. Avoid oversized servings for a healthy balance.

Balanced Meals

Eating a well-rounded meal includes a mix of macronutrients and micronutrients that are important for your body and help you feel full.

It's important to have a mix of foods from various food groups in every meal to get a wide range of nutrients. Whenever you can, go for whole, minimally processed foods and give priority to nutrient-rich choices such as fruits, vegetables, lean proteins, whole grains, and healthy fats.

Remember to always keep in mind these principles as you work towards a healthier lifestyle through clean eating and staying active. Aim to be consistent and moderate in your food choices.

PART II: EMBRACING ACTIVE LIVING

5 THE BENEFITS OF REGULAR EXERCISE

Regular physical exercise is not just important for maintaining good physical health, but it also provides numerous mental and emotional advantages. By including physical activity in your daily schedule, you can enhance every aspect of your overall well-being.

Physical Benefits

- Enhanced Cardiovascular Health: Physical activity boosts heart health and enhances blood flow, lowering the chances of developing heart disease.
- Weight Management: Regular exercise is essential for managing weight effectively as it helps in burning calories and developing lean muscle mass.
- Enhanced Muscle Strength and Stamina: Engaging in strength training helps enhance

muscle strength and stamina, leading to better physical performance and lower chances of injuries.

- Improved Bone Health: Engage in weight-bearing activities such as walking, jogging, and resistance training to enhance your bone health. These exercises are effective in building and preserving bone health.
- Increased Flexibility and Range of Motion: Stretching exercises can enhance your flexibility and range of motion, which in turn helps to minimize the chances of getting injured and promotes better posture.

Mental Benefits

- Stress Reduction: Regular physical activity can lead to a decrease in stress levels by stimulating the production of endorphins. These natural chemicals help to alleviate stress and enhance a sense of calmness and overall happiness.
- Enhanced Well-Being: Engaging in consistent exercise can help reduce feelings of depression and anxiety, leading to a better mood and increased self-confidence.
- Boosted Cognitive Function: Working out enhances your brain function, improves your memory, focus, and decision-making skills.
- Enhancing Sleep Quality: Engaging in regular physical activity can significantly improve sleep quality and aid in managing insomnia and other sleep disorders.

Emotional Benefits

- Increased Energy and Vitality: Regular physical activity boosts energy levels and decreases fatigue, leading to enhanced vitality and overall well-being.
- Boosted Confidence: Achieving fitness goals and improving physical performance can boost self-confidence and self-esteem.
- Sense of Achievement: Accomplishing your set fitness goals will give you feelings of accomplishment and fulfillment, which will in turn enhance your motivation and determination.

How Exercise Enhances Clean Eating

Exercising regularly and clean eating work together to enhance overall health and wellness.

Appetite Regulation

Regular exercise plays a crucial role in balancing appetite hormones like ghrelin and leptin, resulting in better appetite management and a reduced desire for unhealthy foods. This can greatly assist you in adhering to a healthy eating regimen and prevent you from eating excessively.

Better Nutrient Absorption

Engaging in consistent exercise boosts blood flow and nutrient distribution in your body, leading to better absorption of vital nutrients from your meals. This guarantees that your body reaps the full advantages of the nutrient-dense foods that you eat while following a healthy eating regimen.

Improved Metabolism

Working out can speed up your metabolism, making your body burn calories faster and efficiently turn food into energy. This can help in preventing weight gain, especially when paired with a healthy diet centered around whole, nutrient-dense foods.

Stress Reduction

Regular physical activity is an effective way to alleviate stress, as it decreases the production of stress hormones such as cortisol and encourages a sense of calm. By doing so, it can help prevent excessive eating caused by stress and emotional triggers, thereby promoting healthy eating habits.

Maintenance of Lean Muscle Mass

Regularly engaging in strength training exercises is beneficial for both your overall health and metabolism as it helps you maintain and develop lean muscle mass. Additionally, incorporating protein-rich foods into your clean eating diet provides the essential ingredients needed for muscle repair and growth, which further enhances the positive effects of exercise.

Adding regular exercise to your daily schedule can boost the benefits of healthy eating and improve your general health and wellness. In the upcoming section, we'll delve into discovering the perfect workouts that suit your objectives and likes, so you can fully experience the advantages of staying active.

6 FINDING THE RIGHT EXERCISE FOR YOU

It's important to mix things up when it comes to working out. A balanced fitness regimen usually consists of three main forms of exercise.

Cardiovascular Exercise (Cardio)

Engaging in cardiovascular exercise, commonly known as "cardio," involves physical activities that increase your heart rate and breathing rate. Activities like brisk walking, running, cycling, swimming, dancing, and aerobics fall under this category. Cardio workouts are beneficial for improving your cardiovascular health and burning calories..

Strength Training

Strength training, which is also referred to as resistance training or weight training, focuses on enhancing strength, endurance, and muscle mass. You can achieve this by using free weights, weight machines, resistance bands, or even your own body weight. These exercises target different muscle groups, land lead to improvements in your body composition, bone density, and metabolism.

Flexibility and Mobility

Flexibility and mobility exercises are designed to enhance the range of motion in your joints and increase your body flexibility. Some examples of these exercises include stretching, yoga, Pilates, and tai chi. By incorporating these exercises into your routine, you can reduce your risk of injury, alleviate any muscle stiffness, and enhance your posture and balance. Remember to always begin your workout with light stretching to prevent any potential injuries.

Choosing Activities You Enjoy

Finding exercises that you genuinely like and are excited to do is essential for staying consistent with your workout routine. Take into account these aspects when selecting your physical activities:

Personal Preferences

Consider the activities that bring you joy and make you happy. If you enjoy nature, try hiking, biking, or gardening. If you like being around others, consider joining fitness classes or team sports. Keep trying out new activities until you discover what you are most comfortable with.

Fitness Goals

Think about your fitness objectives and how various activities can assist you in reaching them. If your aim is to boost your cardiovascular health, concentrate on cardio exercises such as running or swimming. If you are looking to increase strength and muscle mass, include strength training workouts in your regimen. Select activities that match your goals and preferences.

Accessibility and Convenience

Make sure to select activities that are easily accessible and convenient for you. If you have a busy schedule or limited resources, try to find activities that you can easily do at home or in your local area. Take into account factors such as cost, location, and the availability of equipment when choosing your exercise options.

Creating a Balanced Exercise Routine

Make sure your workout plan includes a mix of

exercises that focus on various fitness goals. Stick to these tips to develop a comprehensive routine:

Include Cardio, Strength Training, and Flexibility Exercises

Make sure to incorporate all three types of exercise into your daily routine to promote your cardiovascular health, build your muscle strength, and enhance your flexibility. Try to vary your activities throughout the week to keep your workouts engaging and to maximize their effectiveness.

Set Realistic Goals

Make sure you establish clear and measurable objectives for your workout regimen. These could include enhancing your stamina, lifting more weight, or enhancing your flexibility. Divide your goals into smaller milestones and keep a record of your progress as time goes by.

Prioritize Consistency

It's important to stay consistent with your exercise routine in order to see results. Make sure to schedule regular workouts throughout your week and prioritize exercise as a non-negotiable part of your daily routine. Strive for at least 150 minutes of moderate-intensity cardio or 75 minutes of vigorous-intensity cardio each week, in addition to incorporating strength training and flexibility exercises on two or more days.

Listen to Your Body

Be mindful of how your body is responding to exercise. If you feel any pain or discomfort, make sure to adjust or stop the activity and seek advice from a healthcare provider if necessary. Pay attention to your body's cues and make changes to your routine to avoid injuries and support your recovery.

––––––––––––––––––

Trying out various forms of exercise, picking activities that bring you joy, and establishing a well-rounded routine with cardio, strength training, and flexibility workouts can help boost your fitness levels, improve your overall health, and lead to a more vibrant and active life..

7 GETTING STARTED WITH FITNESS

Congratulations on taking this first step toward a healthier lifestyle! In this chapter, we will explore the fundamental elements of beginning your fitness adventure. From establishing achievable objectives to discovering workouts suitable for beginners and maintaining motivation and consistency, we will address everything to ensure you start your fitness routine with confidence and excitement.

Setting Realistic Fitness Goals

It is essential to establish practical fitness objectives in order to achieve long-term success. Although it may be tempting to strive for dramatic changes overnight, sustainable progress is based on attainable milestones.

Begin by evaluating your current fitness level and

determining the areas you wish to enhance. Whether it involves improving endurance, building strength, or losing weight, ensure that your goals are specific, measurable, achievable, relevant, and time-bound (SMART).

Divide larger goals into smaller, actionable steps, and take pleasure in celebrating each milestone you reach. Always remember, progress is progress, regardless of its size.

Beginner-Friendly Workouts

Starting a fitness journey might seem overwhelming, especially if you're new to working out. However, there's no need to worry because there are numerous beginner-friendly workouts that are specifically designed to help you ease into physical activity gradually.

Begin with low-impact exercises such as walking, swimming, or cycling to enhance your cardiovascular endurance without straining your joints too much. Integrate strength training into your routine by incorporating bodyweight exercises like squats, lunges, push-ups, and planks to enhance muscle tone and functional strength.

Try out various activities to discover what you enjoy

the most, whether it's yoga, Pilates, or dance fitness classes. The important thing is to engage in activities that you find enjoyable and can sustain in the long run.

Tips for Staying Motivated and Consistent

Maintaining a fitness routine can be quite challenging, especially when it comes to staying motivated and consistent. To assist you in staying on track, here are a few helpful tips:

1. Set Clear Intentions:Take some time to define why you want to make this change and keep those reasons in mind whenever your motivation starts to fade.

2. Find an Accountability Partner: Having someone, be it a friend, family member, or fitness buddy, to keep you on track can offer the encouragement and drive you require.

3. Spice It Up: Add some variety to your workouts by exploring different activities, classes, or workout routines. This will help you stay engaged and avoid boredom.

4. Plan Your Workouts: Give your workouts the importance they deserve by scheduling them in your calendar. Treating them like appointments will help you prioritize exercise and eliminate any excuses.

5. Track Your Progress: Keep a workout journal or use

fitness apps to monitor your progress and celebrate your accomplishments as you go.

6. Treat Yourself: Establish a reward structure for achieving goals or maintaining a regular fitness regimen. Indulge in something you love, such as a spa treatment, new workout gear, or a nutritious meal at your favorite restaurant.

Remember, staying consistent is the key to reaching your fitness objectives. Enjoy the process, show yourself some patience, and acknowledge every little progress you make.

By staying dedicated, persistent, and having a positive attitude, you will soon experience the amazing impact of regular physical activity on your physical health, mental well-being, and overall quality of life.

So, put on your sneakers, channel your inner athlete, and let's start moving towards a healthier, happier version of yourself!

8 INTEGRATING MOVEMENT INTO DAILY LIFE

In this chapter, we will delve into effective techniques to effortlessly incorporate movement into your everyday schedule. Whether it's finding ways to include physical activity in your daily tasks, overcoming obstacles to an active lifestyle, or discovering enjoyable ways to stay fit beyond the gym, you'll gain valuable insights on making fitness an essential component of your life.

Incorporating Physical Activity into Your Daily Activities

You don't have to limit your physical activity to workouts at the gym. There are so many chances to add movement into your day, even while doing daily tasks. Here are a few easy ways to include more activity in your daily life:

1. **Choose the Stairs**: Whenever you have the option, go for the stairs instead of the elevator. It's a great way to incorporate some cardio into your day and give your lower body a good workout.

2. **Opt for Walking or Biking**: If it's possible, try walking or biking to your workplace, school, or when running errands instead of relying on driving. Not only will this increase your daily activity levels, but it will also help reduce your carbon footprint.

3. **Stand Up and Get Moving**: Don't let long periods of sitting get the best of you. Take regular breaks by standing up and moving around every hour. You can even set a timer to remind yourself to stretch, take a walk, or do a quick set of exercises.

4. **Stay Active**: If you can't walk or bike, consider parking further from your destination or getting off public transportation a few stops early to increase your daily steps.

5. **Housework Workout**: Make household chores like vacuuming, mopping, gardening, or washing the car a chance to stay active and burn some calories.

6. **Office Fitness**: Add some simple exercises like leg lifts, calf raises, or desk stretches to your daily routine at work to counteract the downsides of sitting for long periods.

Overcoming Common Barriers to Active Living

It can be challenging to maintain an active lifestyle, even when we have good intentions. Recognizing and tackling these obstacles is key to achieving lasting results. Here are a few common obstacles to staying active and ways to conquer them:

1. **Not Enough Time**: Make physical activity a priority by scheduling it into your daily routine and treating it as essential "me" time. Remember, even short bursts of activity throughout the day can make a difference.

2. **Lack of Motivation**: Discover activities that bring you joy and make you feel great, whether it's dancing, hiking, or participating in a sport. Surround yourself with supportive friends or consider joining a fitness class to stay motivated and accountable.

3. **Unfavorable Weather**: Be prepared for unpredictable weather conditions by investing in suitable gear and having a backup plan for indoor workouts. Embrace outdoor activities like skiing, snowshoeing, or ice skating during the winter months.

4. **Injury or Health Concerns**: Seek guidance from a healthcare professional or certified trainer to create a safe and effective exercise program tailored to your

specific needs and abilities. Focus on low-impact activities and always listen to your body to prevent injuries and promote recovery.

5. **Financial Limitations**: Explore affordable or free options for physical activity, such as community centers, parks, walking trails, or online workout videos. Many fitness apps and websites offer budget-friendly alternatives to expensive gym memberships.

Interesting Ways to Stay Active Outside the Gym

Exercise doesn't have to be boring, you know? There are so many fun activities that can also give you a great workout. You can stay active and have a blast at the same time! Need some inspiration? Here are a few ideas to get your imagination going:

1. Get moving with *dance classes* such as Zumba, salsa, hip-hop, or belly dancing. These classes are not only fun workouts, but they also help boost your mood and confidence.

2. Get out and *explore outside* with thrilling activities like hiking, kayaking or trail running. Nature's beauty will be your companion as you embark on exciting adventures.

3. *Gather your friends* or join a recreational sports

league to enjoy team sports like basketball, soccer, volleyball, or tennis. Not only will you have a blast, but you'll also get a fantastic cardiovascular workout and build camaraderie.

4. Experience the energy and motivation of *group fitness classes* such as spinning, kickboxing, boot camp, or yoga. With an encouraging instructor and lively music, you'll be so engrossed that you won't even realize you're exercising.

5. Engage in *active hobbies* that keep you on the move, like gardening, photography or birdwatching. These hobbies not only provide physical activity but also stimulate your creativity and enhance your mental well-being.

———————————

Finding activities that you love and that effortlessly blend into your daily routine is crucial for maintaining a sustainable fitness regimen.

Whether it's opting for the stairs over the elevator, participating in a dance class, or embarking on a hike with your buddies, every small action contributes to enhancing your overall well-being and energy.

So, seize the chances to incorporate more movement

into your day and enjoy the numerous advantages of an active lifestyle.

PART III: SUSTAINABLE HABITS FOR LONG-TERM SUCCESS

9 MINDFUL EATING AND ACTIVE LIVING

Let's dive into how mindfulness, eating habits, and physical activity are all interconnected in this chapter. By grasping the importance of mindfulness in eating and exercising, along with picking up useful strategies to incorporate mindfulness into your daily life, you can boost your overall health and develop a better relationship with food and fitness.

The Role of Mindfulness in Eating and Exercising

Being fully present and engaged in the moment, without judgment or distraction, is what mindfulness is all about. When you bring this practice to your meals and workouts, you can truly transform your experience and results.

When it comes to eating, practicing mindful eating means being fully present and aware of the sensory experience. This includes savoring the taste, texture, and smell of your food, as well as tuning in to your hunger and fullness cues. By being mindful while eating, you can effectively regulate your appetite, avoid overeating, and truly enjoy every bite.

When it comes to exercising, practicing mindfulness involves being completely in the moment and aware of your body and movements during physical activity. By focusing on the sensations of movement, breath, and muscle engagement, you can enhance your performance, reduce the risk of injury, and strengthen the mind-body connection.

Techniques for Mindful Eating

Practicing mindful eating has the power to completely change your connection with food and enable you to make better choices for your health. Give these techniques a try:

- Savor Each Bite: Take your time to fully chew every mouthful and relish the delicious flavors of your meal. Pause between bites and immerse yourself in the entire sensory experience of eating.

- Listen to Your Body: Pay close attention to your body's signals of hunger and fullness, allowing them to guide your eating habits. Eat when you're genuinely hungry and stop when you feel satisfied, rather than relying on outside influences or emotional triggers.

- Avoid Distractions: Reduce distractions such as television, mobile phones, or computers during meals to fully concentrate on your food and the signals from your body. Establish a calm and peaceful atmosphere that promotes mindful eating.

- Cultivate Thankfulness: Prior to every meal, pause for a moment to express gratitude for the nourishing food in front of you and the chance to provide nourishment for your body and soul.

- Tune in to Your Body: Have faith in your body's innate wisdom and respect its cravings and preferences without any judgment. Opt for foods that leave you feeling energized, satisfied, and well-nourished.

Incorporating Mindfulness into Your Fitness

Routine

Incorporating mindfulness into your fitness routine can truly enhance your overall experience. Not only does it improve your eating habits, but it also adds a new level of enrichment to your workouts. Let's explore how you can bring mindfulness into your exercise regimen:

- Set an Intention: Before starting your workout, establish a goal to direct your focus and drive. Whether it's enhancing strength, boosting flexibility, or simply enjoying in the act of moving, allow your goal shape your workout.

- Concentrate on your breath: Use your breath as a grounding tool to remain in the present moment while exercising. Be mindful of the pace of your breath and synchronize it with your movements to establish a feeling of comfort.

- Be aware of sensations: Pay attention to the sensations in your body as you exercise, identifying areas of tension, discomfort, or comfort. Make adjustments to your movements as needed to respect your body's requirements and prevent injuries.

- Engage in Mindful Movement: View exercise as a way to practice mindfulness and be fully present in the moment. Whether you're doing yoga, tai chi or simply walking, use each movement as a chance to connect with your body and surroundings.

- Show Appreciation: After your workout, pause to show gratitude for your body's strength, flexibility, and mobility. Recognize the hard work you've done and the positive impact it has had on your well-being.

By integrating mindfulness into your meals and workouts, you'll develop a greater understanding of your body and mind, and how they are connected. Take your time, focus, and appreciate every moment to turn ordinary tasks into enriching moments that feed your body, mind, and spirit.

10 OVERCOMING CHALLENGES AND SETBACKS

Now let us look into techniques to conquer common hurdles and setbacks that might come up while embarking on your path towards healthy eating and living an active lifestyle.

Whether it's dealing with cravings and emotional eating, staying committed to your fitness objectives, or effectively managing stress, you will acquire the skills to overcome obstacles with unwavering determination and resilience.

Dealing with Cravings and Emotional Eating

Giving in to your cravings and emotional eating can throw off your progress towards a healthier lifestyle, no matter how determined you are. Whether you're hit with a sudden desire for something sugary or you find yourself reaching for food when you're stressed, it's important to find ways to deal with these obstacles.

- Pinpoint Triggers: Take note of what triggers your cravings or emotional eating. It could be boredom, stress, sadness, or social situations. Once you identify these triggers, you can work on finding healthier ways to deal with them.

- Embrace Mindful Eating: Slow down and listen to your body's signals of hunger and fullness before grabbing a snack. Determine if you're eating because you're truly hungry or if it's an emotional response, then choose foods that nourish both your body and mind.

- Opt for Healthier Options: Fill your kitchen with nutritious alternatives to your usual comfort foods, like fresh fruits, nuts or a piece of dark chocolate. Select foods that satisfy your cravings while still aligning with your health goals.

- Distract Yourself: When you feel the urge to eat emotionally, distract yourself with activities that don't involve food, such as taking a stroll, practicing relaxation techniques, or pursuing a hobby. Redirect your attention towards things that bring you happiness and contentment.

Staying on Track with Fitness Goals

To stay on track towards your fitness goals, it's important to have dedication and resilience when faced with challenges. Here are some tips to help you stay on track:

- Set Achievable Goals: Divide your fitness goals into smaller, realistic targets to monitor your progress and celebrate milestones as you go. Concentrate on things within your control, like working out a specific number of days each week or gradually increasing your workout intensity.

- Develop a Routine: Create a regular exercise routine that suits your timetable and preferences. Consider physical activity as a non-negotiable part of your day, just like brushing your teeth or having meals.

- Seek Support: Get the assistance of friends, family, or a workout partner to stay motivated and responsible. Share your objectives, progress, and challenges with people who can provide encouragement and assistance.

- Keep It Interesting: Avoid monotony by changing your workout routines frequently. Include various types of exercises in your routine to keep your body challenged and engaged.

Strategies for Managing Stress and Avoiding Burnout

Stress is a common challenge that can result in burnout if not properly addressed. Here are some effective techniques to effectively handle stress:

- Prioritize Self-Care: Make yourself a priority by incorporating relaxation techniques such as meditation, yoga, deep breathing, or massages into your daily routine. Take breaks to recharge and rejuvenate your mind and body regularly.

- Practice Time Management: Manage your time effectively by organizing your schedule and prioritizing tasks. Break down larger tasks into smaller, more actionable steps, and delegate or eliminate non-essential activities whenever possible to reduce feelings of overwhelm and stress.

- Establish Boundaries: Set boundaries to protect your time, energy, and well-being. Learn to say no to commitments that don't align with your priorities and values, and don't hesitate to ask for help when you need it.

- Seek Support: Don't hesitate to seek support from friends, family members, or a mental health professional during challenging times. Rely on your network for encouragement when you need it.

———————————

Remember that setbacks are a normal part of any journey, and each obstacle you conquer builds your determination and brings you closer to your aspirations. Stay determined, stay strong, and continue progressing towards a healthier and happier version of yourself.

11 BUILDING A SUPPORT SYSTEM

Starting on a path towards healthy eating and regular exercise may be challenging without a reliable support network. Social support offers emotional backing, useful tips, and responsibility, which can keep you inspired and dedicated to achieving your objectives.

Research shows that individuals who have a strong support system are more likely to accomplish and sustain their health and fitness objectives. This chapter explores the crucial significance of social support in your journey towards wellness, and provides effective techniques for establishing and nurturing a resilient support network.

Benefits of Social Support

1. Motivation and Encouragement: Having a strong support system of friends and family can provide the motivation and encouragement you need, especially when facing difficult times.

2. Accountability: When you share your goals with others, it creates a sense of accountability that helps you stay committed to healthy habits.

3. Shared Knowledge: Being part of a supportive network allows you to tap into a wealth of knowledge, receive valuable advice, and gain practical tips to help you succeed.

4. Emotional Support: Going through lifestyle changes can be emotionally challenging, but having people to talk to and share your experiences with can help alleviate stress and promote mental well-being.

5. Celebration of Successes: Celebrating your milestones and achievements with others not only boosts your sense of accomplishment but also keeps you motivated to continue striving for success.

Finding Community and Accountability

Finding a group of people who have similar health and fitness goals can offer valuable encouragement and motivation. Here are some tips for connecting with others who share your goals:

Join Local Groups

- Fitness Classes: Engage in fitness classes held at your nearby gym or community center. Group workout sessions not only help you stay fit, but also foster a sense of togetherness and shared objectives.

- Nutrition Workshops: Take part in workshops or cooking classes that emphasize healthy eating and nutrition. These gatherings are an excellent opportunity to connect with individuals who share your passion for clean eating.

- Sports Teams: Become a member of a sports team or recreational league to enjoy physical exercise and social interaction at the same time. It's a fantastic way to stay active while making new friends.

Online Communities

- Social Media Groups: Connect with like-minded individuals by becoming a member of Facebook groups or Instagram communities focused on clean eating and active living. Participate in conversations, exchange helpful tips, and find support from others who are on a similar journey.

- Fitness Apps: Use fitness apps that provide community features, allowing you to connect with fellow users, share your progress, and take part in exciting challenges.

- Online Forums: Explore online forums such as Reddit and specialized health platforms to engage in discussions about nutrition, fitness, and overall well-being. These platforms provide a space for you to connect with others who share similar interests and goals.

Accountability Partners

- Friends and Family: Get support from a close friend or family member who has similar goals. Stay connected and engaged with each other to stay on track.

- Workplace Wellness Programs: Take advantage of workplace wellness initiatives that promote healthy habits. Engage with coworkers who are also striving for wellness.

- Professional Support: Seek assistance from a health coach, nutritionist, or personal trainer for professional guidance and accountability.

How to Inspire and Support Others on Their Journey

Helping others on their health and fitness path can bring you great satisfaction and can also strengthen your dedication to staying healthy. Here are a few ways to motivate and back up those in your circle:

Lead by Example

- Display Healthy Habits: Show your dedication to maintaining a nutritious diet and staying physically active by leading by example. Your commitment has the potential to inspire others to adopt similar habits.

- Share Your Successes: Share your triumphs and the positive outcomes you've encountered as a result of your lifestyle choices. Personal stories can serve as motivators.

Offer Practical Support

- Meal Prep and Cook Together: Extend an invitation to your friends or family members to join you in preparing nutritious meals in advance. This collaborative effort can add a touch of enjoyment and learning to the process.

- Workout Partners: Encourage others to join you during exercise sessions or engaging in physical activities. By working out together, you can infuse a sense of fun to fitness.

- Share Resources: Share your favorite books (like this one, hopefully), recipes, apps, or websites that have helped you in your own journey. By offering valuable resources, you can inspire and empower others to take proactive steps towards their goals.

Encourage and Celebrate

- Give Encouragement: Share words of support and praise when others make positive choices or achieve set goals. Offering positive feedback can uplift their spirits and inspire them to keep going.

- Celebrate Milestones: Recognize and celebrate the accomplishments of those in your circle, regardless of their size. Celebrating achievements can strengthen their determination and validate their hard work.

Be a Supportive Listener

- Listen Without Judgment: Provide a safe environment where others can freely express their struggles and successes. By listening without judgment, you can make them feel heard and encouraged.

- Offer Empathy : Recognize that everyone's journey is distinct and may come with unique challenges. Instead of giving unwanted advice, offer empathy and understanding to foster a supportive atmosphere.

Keep in mind, your encouragement has the power to motivate others to start their journey towards improved health, sparking a chain reaction of positive transformation.

12 TRACKING PROGRESS AND CELEBRATING SUCCESS

Nutrition Tracking

Monitoring your nutrition is a great way to stay accountable and pinpoint areas where you can make improvements. These are some approaches you can take:

- Food Diaries: By writing down everything you eat and drink in a daily food diary, you can gain insight into your eating patterns and make necessary changes. Make sure you include portion sizes, meal times, and how hungry or full you feel.

- Mobile Apps: Nutrition tracking apps such as MyFitnessPal, Lose It! and Cronometer make the process easier with their wide food databases and nutrient details. These apps allow you scan barcodes, log meals, and monitor your nutrient intake.

- Picture Evidence: Snap photos of your meals as a quick and visual way to keep tabs on your eating habits. This method can also help you gauge portion sizes and the variety of foods you're consuming.

Fitness Tracking

Keeping track of your fitness journey helps you stay motivated and ensure you're achieving your fitness goals. Here are some effective ways to do so:

- Use Fitness Apps and Wearables: Apps such as Fitbit, Strava, and Apple Health, as well as wearable devices, can monitor your daily activities, workouts, steps, heart rate, and more. These tools offer detailed data to help you analyze your fitness progress.

- Maintain Workout Logs: Keep a workout log to document specifics of your exercise routines, such as the type of workout, duration, intensity, and any personal records or milestones accomplished. This will enable you to monitor progress in your strength, endurance, and overall fitness.

- Take Progress Photos and Measurements: Regularly taking photos and measuring your body can give you a visual representation of your progress. Measure areas like your waist, hips, chest, and limbs, and compare them over time to observe physical transformations.

Setting Milestones and Celebrating Achievements

Setting Milestones

Divide your long-term objectives into smaller, achievable milestones to make the journey more manageable and inspiring. Here's how to establish effective milestones:

- Be Specific and Measurable: Make sure each milestone is clear and quantifiable. For instance, instead of a broad goal like "get in shape," set a specific objective like "complete a 5K in less than 40 minutes" or "shed 8 pounds in three months."

- Be Realistic and Attainable: Your milestones should be challenging yet realistic. Attaining feasible targets helps you sustain motivation and minimizes your chances of feeling disheartened.

- Be Time-Bound: Attach a deadline to each milestone. This creates a sense of urgency and helps you concentrate on your progress.

Celebrating Achievements

Recognizing and celebrating your accomplishments, no matter how small, is essential for maintaining motivation. Here are a few ways to celebrate your milestones:

- Treat Yourself: Indulge in something enjoyable that aligns with your healthy lifestyle. It could be a new workout gear, a rejuvenating massage, or a special outing that brings you joy.

- Share Your Success: Spread the word about your achievements with friends, family, or a supportive online community. Their encouragement and acknowledgment can uplift your spirits and keep you motivated.

- Reflect on Your Journey: Take a moment to look back on how far you've come and the obstacles you've conquered. Writing about your progress in a journal can give you a sense of fulfillment and inspire you to keep pushing forward.

Adjusting Goals and Plans for Continued Growth

Reassessing and Adjusting Goals

As you progress, it's important to regularly reassess your goals and make adjustments to ensure continued growth and improvement. Here's how to effectively adjust your goals:

- Evaluate Progress: Periodically review your progress towards your goals. Assess what's working, what's not, and whether you're moving in the right direction.

- Set New Challenges: Once you achieve a milestone, set new, more challenging goals to push yourself further. This prevents complacency and keeps you motivated.

- Adapt to Changes: Life circumstances, health conditions, and personal priorities can change over time. Be flexible and adapt your goals to align with your current situation and capabilities.

Updating Plans and Strategies

To maintain long-term success, you need to

constantly update your plans and strategies. Here are a few suggestions to ensure your plans remain dynamic:

- Embrace Variety: Injecting variety into your workouts and meal plans is key to avoiding boredom and staying motivated. Experiment with different exercises or recipes to keep things interesting and challenging.

- Seek Feedback: Regularly seek input from fitness trainers, nutritionists, or supportive peers. Their feedback can help you fine-tune your approach and overcome any obstacles you may encounter along the way.

- Stay Informed: Stay up-to-date with the latest research and trends in nutrition and fitness. This knowledge will not only inspire new strategies but also enhance your overall plan, ensuring you are always on top of your game.

As you look back on your accomplishments and embrace fresh obstacles, keep in mind that each progress you make is a triumph worth commemorating. Continue to move ahead with excitement, knowing that your dedication to a healthier way of life is bringing you priceless benefits.

CONCLUSION

As we come to the end of this book, let's take a moment to recap the earlier essential points we've covered in this journey:

- **Principles of Clean Eating**: Focus on whole, unprocessed foods and nutrient-dense options. Clean eating is all about fueling your body with natural, wholesome goodness.

- **Macronutrients and Micronutrients**: Knowing the importance of proteins, carbs, fats, vitamins, and minerals helps you make smart food choices to maintain your overall well-being.

- **Portion Control and Balanced Meals**: By practicing portion control and creating balanced meals, you can ensure you're getting all the essential nutrients without overeating, supporting a healthy weight and optimal body function.

- **Benefits of Clean Eating and Active Living**: From increased energy and improved digestion to better mental health and reduced inflammation, adopting this lifestyle can bring about a wide range of positive changes.

- **Practical Strategies and Recipes**: Equipped with meal planning advice, pantry essentials, and tasty recipes, this book has given you the building blocks you need to incorporate clean eating and active living into your everyday life.

Encouragement for Continued Commitment to Health

Transitioning to a clean eating and active lifestyle is a big step towards improving your health and well-being. It's important to keep in mind that this journey isn't about being perfect, but rather about consistently making mindful choices that align with your health goals.

Take the time to celebrate your progress, no matter how small, and stay dedicated to the habits that promote your well-being.

There will be obstacles and setbacks along the way, but don't let them discourage you. Instead, view them as opportunities to learn and become even stronger.

Surround yourself with a supportive community, whether it's friends, family, or individuals who share your health aspirations. Remember, every positive decision you make is an investment in your health and future.

My Final Thoughts

Living a nourished and thriving life extends beyond the food you consume and the exercises you engage in. It involves adopting a holistic approach to wellness that encompasses your physical, mental, and emotional well-being.

By embracing a clean eating regimen and an active lifestyle, you are laying the groundwork for a life brimming with vitality, energy, and happiness.

As you progress, continue to explore new foods, experiment with various physical activities, and deepen your understanding of your body and its requirements. Remain curious and receptive to new experiences that enhance your overall health and well-being.

Your journey towards a healthier lifestyle is an ongoing process, and each step you take brings you closer to the vibrant life you deserve.

I sincerely appreciate your decision to embark on this journey with "Eat Well to Live Well." May the knowledge and resources you have acquired empower you to live your healthiest and most fulfilling life.

ABOUT THE AUTHOR

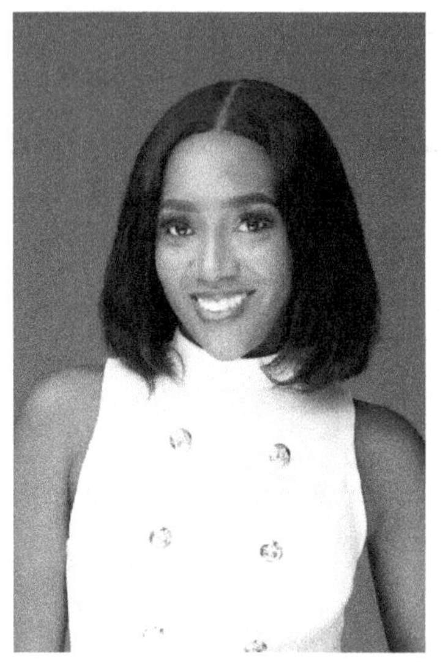

Dr. Nimi Aworinde is a dedicated medical doctor with a profound passion for preventive health and wellness. Her commitment to enhancing the lives of others through proper nutrition and active living stems from her deep belief in the power of food as medicine.

With years of experience in the medical field, she has seen firsthand how clean eating and active living can transform lives, and she is devoted to sharing this message with a broader audience. Her empathetic approach and dedication to teaching make her a trusted and beloved figure in her community.

In **"Eat Well to Live Well: The Essential Guide to Clean Eating and Active Living"**, Dr. Aworinde combines her medical expertise with her passion for nutrition to provide you with a comprehensive and easy-to-understand guide that empowers you to take control of your health and live your best life. Through this book, she hopes to inspire a healthier, happier world, one meal at a time.

She shares her insights on nutrition, health, and wellness through articles posted on her blog at www.vitaliciousvibes.blogspot.com.